TEMPLE TALK

TAKING CARE OF YOUR BODY, THE TEMPLE OF YOUR SOUL

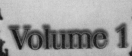

Volume 1

Oxygenation, Assimilation & Elimination

JEANNIE CALLIS

Human GRoth gbzmone

Unless otherwise indicated, all Scripture quotations are taken from the King James Version of the Bible.

Temple Talk
ISBN 0-9659640-0-0
Copyright © Jeannie Callis
P. O. Box 152
Argyle, Texas 76226
Published August, 1997

TABLE OF CONTENTS

❧

DEDICATION

This work is dedicated
to the
GREAT MASTER
whose grace, body and blood
made this book possible.

In loving memory of my late husband,
Reverend Gail Dwain Callis and five deceased
children, whose lives and deaths have greatly
inspired me in writing this book. I would also like
to say how blessed I am for my two sons and their
children. I thank all others who have had a part in
the sowing of this seed into your life.

God is the *Healer* of the body;
we are the *keeper* of the body.

Read 2 Kings 20:1-7.

I'M SPECIAL

I'm Special . . .
>In all the world there's nobody like me.
>Nobody has my smile.
>Nobody has my eyes, nose, hair or voice.

I'm Special . . .
>No one laughs like me or cries like me.
>No one sees things just as I do.
>No one reacts just as I would react.

I'm Special . . .
>I'm the only one in all creation who has my
>set of abilities.
>My unique combination of gifts, talents and
>abilities are an original symphony.

I'm Special . . .
>I'm rare.
>And in all rarity there is great value.
>I need not imitate others. I will accept – yes
>celebrate – my differences.

I'm Special . . .
>And I'm beginning to see that God made me
>special for a very special purpose.
>God has a job for me that no one else can do as
>well as I do.
>Out of all the applicants, only one is faithful.
>That is me.

Because . . . . .I'm Special!

Author Unknown

TEMPLE TALK

▶ God is the Owner of the Temple.
We are the Trustees, in charge of care and
maintenance.

▶ Practical advice for well-being — our physical
and spiritual health.

▶ The central theme of this book is that each of us
is personally responsible for our own health.

▶ Practical suggestions for taking care of your own
Temple by using the three natural principles for
a healthy immune system — essential oxygen,
assimilation and elimination.

~ Proverbs 4:7 ~

**Wisdom is the *principal* thing;
therefore get wisdom: and with all thy
getting *get understanding*.**

BIOGRAPHICAL SKETCH

JEANNIE CALLIS

by Jocelyn W. Alexander

Jeannie Callis is a remarkable woman whose entire life has been of service, and of *creating solutions* to innumerable types of life situations.

Jeannie was born the fifth child of seven children to farmers that did share cropping and traveled and worked other people's fields. Even as a small child, Jeannie was inquisitive about *healing methods* – whether for a plant, animal or person. She grew up in a family devoted to hard physical work and to doing their best in solving their own problems. There was very little money, so that they learned to use their own resources; and home remedies were used for healing family illnesses.

Jeannie was sexually molested as a child. Just before her tenth birthday, her parents divorced and she went to live with her father. She cooked, ironed, and learned to plant and can their food. She would get up each morning at about 4:00, build a fire in the wood cook stove and fix breakfast. There were no close neighbors. When her father left for work, she was so frightened out in the woods by herself that she would sit out in the hallway until daylight. She then made the beds and caught the bus to go to school.

All the grades had one teacher, Mrs. Grace. Jeannie packed her own lunch in a big sack so it looked like she had a lot to eat. She would hide in the cloak room and eat her lunch because she did not want the other boys and girls know that she only had a biscuit with syrup to eat. She did not know that you could buy bread.

Her father married a second time. He passed away not long after that. Living with her mother and assisting in the care of a younger brother and sister, she does not recall ever attending church until the age of 17.

Jeannie was never sick as a child, but eagerly learned the remedies she observed being used on others. From the time Jeannie was a little tike in the cotton fields, there was never a period that she didn't have some kind of job or work project. When only seventeen years old, she began working in the mental hospital in Austin, Texas.

She married at age eighteen to a young man she had met in church, who later became a minister, and from then on was involved in ministering to the sick and counseling those in need.

During the next eight years of her life, she miscarried quadruplets, gave birth by cesarean to three other children. She divorced and married him again, then divorced him a second time. While divorced she met and married a man with two children. After being convinced by relatives that you could not have a living husband and be married to another man, the church had the marriage annulled. After resigning herself to just raise her children and live for the Lord, her first husband came back into the picture.

He dedicated himself to the Lord, and she was assured that she would never have a cause to divorce him again. Jeannie's pastor performed her third marriage ceremony to this man. They began to go out into the ministry and build a church. *Her spiritual warfare begun*. Their mentors, those who taught them before they went into the ministry, tried to convince her husband to close the church, that he was not a minister, that he had not been called to God. These circumstances caused her life to become increasingly stressful. Whenever your spouse or your family suffers, you take that on yourself. But Jeannie's philosophy has always been, *"It's not what comes your way, it's how you handle it."*

Her husband took ill. They had built two churches 45 miles apart. He ministered on Wednesday and went into a coma and passed away on Sunday morning, leaving Jeannie with two churches, two homes, four automobiles, two children, $1,200 worth of insurance (not $12,000) to bury him and raise their children. She was left without a shepherd. Her husband was her shepherd. She was a shepherd's wife. After the passing of her husband, she felt like a sheep again, and needed a shepherd. So in searching for a place to worship, she went back to the church where she had met her husband and found out that they had no shepherd there. The shepherd had been put out at that time for adultery.

Under the stress of all of this, *Jeannie suffered a heart attack, and was given six months to live.* Shortly thereafter she had an accident requiring emergency surgery. She accepted this as another challenge – to find a way *to heal herself.* After *fifty-one days in bed,* she began to force herself to get up and gradually regained enough strength to travel to Alaska to stay with her sister, breathe the fresh air, and begin life anew.

It was at this time that she turned her attention towards *helping the physical body* — her own body as well as others.

After four years of more varied work experience and self-healing in Alaska, Jeannie returned to Texas to find she had been illegally denied ownership of her church property. Legal battles ensued, and more stress, bringing another major challenge to Jeannie — *the discovery of breast cancer.* She *refused* chemotherapy and the conventional cancer treatments, and pursued *natural therapies,* primarily *colonics* and a way of *eating* she was not accustomed to.

After six months, there was no trace of cancer in her body, but she was left with a sense of responsibility to share with others her new-found knowledge of the benefits of internal cleansing and natural diet.

From this point came extensive study in the field of colon therapy, polarity, kinesiology, and emergency medical training, and enough certificates of merit to cover the entire wall of a room.

Jeannie opened the Progressive Journey Therapy Center in Brady, Texas in 1980, which marked a significant point in her own progressive journey. Shortly after that, she opened a branch clinic in Midland, Texas and was traveling 200 miles between the two clinics every month.

It became more feasible to have one clinic between the two points, which led to a move to San Angelo, Texas and the opening of a clinic there.

The next move was to Mexico to help Dr. Ray Evers establish a clinic, where she was on 24-hour call to answer and direct any emergency crisis, and teach colonic, hydro and physical therapies.

After the death of Dr. Evers, Jeannie was instrumental in assisting six other colon therapists to begin their own practice. She later helped with the founding of Healing Springs Ranch in Tioga, Texas, before opening her own Life Energizers Clinic in Grand Prairie, Texas. After building a successful business there in a very short time, Jeannie sold the business, so she would be free to travel and teach, thereby reaching more people with whom to share her wisdom and experience.

That's the reason for this book — to assist others in their own health and well-being.

TEMPLE TALK

Taking Care Of The Body
The Temple Of Your Soul

Jeannie Callis intends in no way to force a decision that is not of your own choosing. This is not the *only* way to have health and well-being. It is one way to teach oneself *wisdom* and understanding of the *flow of life* which is *energy in the body.*

1 Corinthians 6:19,20 : *"What? Know ye not that your body is the temple of the Holy Ghost which is in you, which ye have of God, and ye are not your own? For you are bought with a price: therefore glorify God in your body, and in your spirit, which are God's."*

GOD'S NATURAL LAW

When God walked with Adam and Eve in the Garden of Eden, there was no *time* and no *end*; therefore no *death*. God created the *natural law* of the universe, which is health and well-being.

~ Chapter 1 ~

UNDERSTANDING THE BODY'S FUNCTIONS

Understanding the human body is critical to understanding yourself. When you understand more about how nutrition and human functions are so closely interrelated, you will be better equipped to nurture your body into and maintain an excellent state of health.

When we understand *the process* for which the body is actually fed, or not fed and cleansed, we will comprehend the *cause* of the body's malfunctions. Then we can make our own decision as to whether we want to merely cover up the problem by relieving the symptoms, or *change our habits* to properly take care of the body so that it can function as God intended it.

Physical well-being is important for happiness, character, and service. It is impossible for the fatigued to enjoy life as much as a well person. The one who has worn nerves has difficulty in controlling his disposition. The individual with a weak constitution is limited in his service. Health, then, is a vital issue. We need a sound body if we are able to have a spirit able to do its best.

No sooner do we consider this important matter

than a number of difficulties appear that enable us to
see that good health is not so much a heritage as an
achievement. There are many difficulties that confront
us, and we need to be alert to the conditions and the
needs.

It would be impossible here to go into an extensive
discussion of the nature, causes, and results of disease.
We are readily aware of the fact that almost all kinds of
diseases are prevalent *around* us, if not in us, *most of the
time.*

One has to think of the large number suffering from
the major ailments — heart trouble, pneumonia, cancer,
etc. — to realize the ravages of disease. In addition to
these are the many minor troubles resulting from
epidemics, indulgence, overwork, and other causes
which may develop into major problems. Millions of
people in the United States are sick constantly.

THE IMPORTANCE OF THE BRAIN

It is the brain that counts. In order that your brain
may be kept clear, you must keep your body fit and
well.

RECOGNIZE THE SACREDNESS OF THE BODY

Some people are inclined to think of the *spiritual*
phase of life as the only one of worth and therefore
discount the physical.

Christ was a red-blooded man, able to do carpenter work, walk long distances, and drive money changers from the temple. *More than three-fourths of his miracles had to do with healing.*

Paul said, "Your body is a temple (sanctuary) of the Holy Spirit which is in you." (1 Corinthians 6:19.) He considered the body not only as the *abiding* place of the Holy Spirit, but also as a member of Christ (1 Corinthians 6:15), and therefore sacred. Such a viewpoint is necessary if we are to have the right attitude, especially in light of temptations we face today.

UNDERSTAND ITS INFLUENCE ON THE SPIRIT

The body and the soul are very intimately related. There is a definite interaction between the two. Increasingly, modern psychology and medicine are recognizing this fact. This close relationship causes the spiritual aspect of life to be greatly influenced by the physical.

▶ One cannot make as good a speech after a heavy meal as before.

▶ The melancholic person is pessimistic, and the sanguine is optimistic and cheerful.

Life worth living does in part depend on the condition of the *body*. A sound body is needed for a sound mind. You cannot be as good as you might be unless you are as fit as you can be.

This fact being true, the religious person must pay some attention to the physical aspect of life as a part of his stewardship.

Have a physical checkup occasionally; know something about what agrees and what disagrees with you. And take a long look before you develop a habit that may be detrimental to your body.

You should limit your activities, even religious ones, to those that your body can stand.

Dr. J. B. Gambrell once refused to join in a day of fasting, saying that he could work better with his body well-nourished that particular day.

REALIZE THAT HEALTH IS OBTAINABLE

Many people still seem to feel that disease is something mysterious, therefore, beyond the responsibility of man.

DEVELOP A CONSCIENCE ON THE MATTER

It is conceivable to realize the influence of the body on the Spirit and know that health is possible. Frequently people consult doctors and even take the time and money necessary to go through clinics for evaluation, and yet never have a prescription filled or follow any advice given.

Knowledge alone is not an adequate incentive.

There must be a *conviction* on matters of this sort before time and energy will be expended to overcome the evils. Motivation is the supreme problem.

It took a religious motive to keep Joseph pure in Egypt and to enable Daniel to refuse the King's wines.

The spiritual must be made to dominate the physical. Like Paul, we must develop the ideal of keeping our bodies in subjection.

Proverbs 18:4 — *"The spirit of a man will sustain his infirmity; but a wounded spirit who can bear?"*

~ What Does Being Healthy Mean~

Health can be defined several different ways. What does it mean to you.

1. <u>Anglo Saxon Root:</u> Definition - "Hole, sound or whole".

2. <u>World Health Organization:</u> Definition - Complete physical, mental and social well-being, not merely the absence of disease or infirmity.

3. To say you are healthy - if your temperature, blood pressure and the like are all normal.

The problem with that biological variability: what is normal for someone else may be abnormal for you.

In other words, to be healthy, you don't have to measure up to any absolute standards. You just meet the demands of your daily life.

~ Chapter 2 ~

NATURAL PRINCIPLES FOR A HEALTHY IMMUNE SYSTEM

Since it is the natural law for the body to be healthy, an *immune* system developed. As long as one follows the natural principles, the immune system will function properly, giving protection from illness.

There are three factors essential to maintaining a healthy immune system.

▶ **OXYGENATION** – the *process* by which the body utilizes its number one nutrient, *oxygen*.

▶ **ASSIMILATION** – the body's ability to make use of all *nutrients* taken in: oxygen, food, vitamins, minerals, and water.

▶ **ELIMINATION** – the body *ridding itself* of waste matter through the lungs, kidneys, skin, and bowels.

OXYGEN
The Body's
Security System

~ Chapter 3 ~

OXYGENATION

Oxygen is the life giver.
Life is absolutely dependent upon the act of breathing. *"BREATH IS LIFE".* To breath is to live and without breath there is no life.

The infant draws in a long deep breath, *exhales* it in a long wail — its life on earth has begun. The old man gives a faint gasp or ceases to breath — and life is over. From the first breath of the infant to the last gasp of the dying man, it is one long story of *continued* breathing. *Life is but a series of breaths.*

Oxygen is the body's number one nutrient. Deprived of oxygen, the brain at a normal temperature will die or be damaged within 8 to 10 minutes. A drowning victim trapped under cool or cold water can be revived without brain damage when oxygen is quickly restored.

WAYS TO GET ADEQUATE OXYGEN INTO YOUR SYSTEM

▶ THROUGH THE NOSTRILS.

Genesis 2:7 — *"And the Lord God formed man of the dust of the ground, and breathed into his nostrils the breath of life; and man became a living soul."*

One of the first essentials of life is to learn how to breathe through the *nostrils*, and to overcome the common practice of mouth breathing. Man is so constructed that he may breathe either through the mouth or nasal tubes. But it is a matter of vital importance to him *which method he follows;* as one brings health and strength and the other disease and weakness.

Take deep breaths filling up the lower part of the lungs. If the nostrils are narrow slits that pull in and tend to close on the inhale, you are not getting enough oxygen, and are only breathing into the upper chest, and not filling up the lower part of the lungs.

It is the breathing and muscle action that moves the blood. The deeper we breathe, the better *circulation* we have in the body. This is the reason exercise benefits our health so much. *Exercise enables us to take fuller breaths, which brings more oxygen to the blood.* Oxygenated blood eliminates toxins and breeding grounds for parasites.

The body is divided in half. Therefore, the left nostril dominately oxygenates the left brain and the right nostril dominately oxygenates the right brain. When the body is "in balance" the way it was designed, oxygen will be taken in through *both* nostrils. Otherwise, the body's natural instincts will try to alternate sides every hour and a half or so.

When breath is taken through the *mouth*, you will get *less* oxygen to the brain.

The nostrils are two narrow channels containing numerous bristly hairs which serve the purpose of a filter or sieve to *strain the air* of its impurities. These impurities are expelled when the breath is exhaled back through the nostrils — like a fish gulps in dirty water then blows it back out again. The impurities which are stopped and retained by sieves and mucous membranes of the nostrils are thrown out again by the *expelled* breath. One who habitually breathes through the nostrils is not likely to be troubled with clogged or stuffy nostrils.

Not only do the nostrils serve this important purpose, but they also perform an important function in *warming* the breath as it is *inhaled.*

When breath is taken in through *both* nostrils, oxygen will go to the hypothalamus and pituitary gland sending oxygen and its messages to the brain *evenly.* The brain is plugged into the body with all its organs, veins, arteries, tissue cells and bones. This then oxygenates the body properly.

During *inhalation,* the diaphragm (the breathing muscle) contracts and exerts a gentle pressure on the liver, stomach and other organs. This action in connection with the rhythm of the lungs acts as a gentle *massage* of these organs and *stimulates* their actions, and encourages normal functioning. Each inhalation helps in this internal exercise and assists in the normal circulation of nutrients to the organs, promoting proper *elimination of waste.*

LUNGS

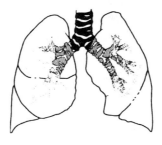

Respiration is a life-supporting process whereby oxygen from incoming air enters the blood and carbon dioxide, a waste gas from the metabolism of food, is *exhaled.* The *lungs* are paired organs in the chest that carry on *respiration.*

Air enters the lungs when the diaphragm, a strong muscle *under* the lungs, forcibly lowers and enlarges the chest cavity in which the lungs are suspended. This causes the lungs to expand and the air to fill the enlarged lungs. When the diaphragm (breathing muscle) relaxes, the lungs contract and the air is forced out. In times of greater oxygen need, the rib cage can also expand, further enlarging the chest cavity for *greater* air intake. A healthy adult can draw in about 3.3 to 4.9 liters (about 200 to 300 cu in) of air at a single breath, but at rest, only about 5 percent of this volume is used. Lungs also excrete water as *gas,* store glycogen (a complex carbohydrate), and *filter out* incoming organisms and dangerous particles via hairs called *cilia.*

Now, this information seems a little detailed and "medical," but it is too important to overlook.

The exchange of gases takes place when air reaches the *alveoli*. These small sacs are only one cell thick, and they are surrounded by *blood capillaries* that are also only one cell thick. Air *diffuses* through these cells into the capillary blood, which carries the oxygen-rich air *to the heart* to be distributed throughout the body. In the alveoli, at the same time, gaseous carbon dioxide diffuses from the blood into the lung and is *expired*.

In the adult human, each lung is 25 to 30 cm (10 to 12 inches) long. The two lungs are separated by a structure which contains the heart, trachea, esophagus, and blood vessels. They are covered by a protective membrane called the *pulmonary pleura*, which is separated from the *parietal* pleura — a similar membrane on the chest wall — by a lubricating fluid. *Inhaled* air passes through the trachea which divides into two tubes called *bronchi*. Each bronchus leads to one lung. Within the lungs, the bronchi subdivide into *bronchioles* which give rise to *alveolar ducts*. These *end* in sacs called *alveoli*.

Bottom line? *Fill those lungs with oxygen!*

▶ THROUGH THE BLOOD

Leviticus 17:11 — *"For the life of the flesh is in the blood."*

The blood contains *oxygen* which the cells need in order for the body to function without symptoms of tiredness, sickness, and disease.

Blood is the life stream of the body, affecting every cell and system we possess.

There are *three* main types of cells in the bloodstream — *red cells, white cells and plasma.*

Red blood cells are the most numerous, making up about 40% of the total blood volume. The red blood cells are oxygenated and are perfectly *round* in shape. *White* blood cells and platelets make up about 5% of the blood volume. They are part of the body's *defense* system and help keep the red cells *protected* and each organ defended against disease. The red cells have a *positive* charge while the white cells have a negative charge — thus keeping them from sticking together. The remaining half of the blood is composed of *plasma* — a sticky substance made up of approximately 95% water and 5% plasma.

Un-oxygenated and *under*-nourished red blood cells will become oblong and odd shaped. They can clump together, preventing the positive and negative charged blood cells from giving us life more abundantly.

John 10:10 — *". . . I come that they might have life, and that they might have it more abundantly."*

Our blood uses enzyme-enriched hormones to absorb oxygen in the lungs and carry the oxygen to every body part.

Unless fresh air in sufficient quantities reaches the lungs, the stream of *venous* blood cannot be purified. Consequently, not only is the body robbed of nourishment, but the *waste* products which should have been destroyed are *returned* to the circulation and poison the system.

If one does not breathe in a sufficient quantity of air, the vital work of the blood cannot be carried out. The result is that the body is insufficiently nourished and disease occurs, or a state of imperfect health is experienced. When properly exposed to air in the lungs, the blood not only has its impurities consumed and parts with its noxious carbonic acid gas, but it also takes up and absorbs quality oxygen that it carries to all parts of the body.

When blood cannot circulate to the cells that make up this physical temple, or when the blood is toxic or *unoxygenated*, the cells do not get fed or cleansed; thus they begin to die *prematurely*. When these cells begin to die in some areas of the body, it is just a matter of time before symptoms are experienced.

▶ **THROUGH THE SKIN**

The skin helps keep the body cool. When temperatures rise, the skin radiates heat flow and provides a surface for the evaporation of sweat. Sweat is also known as perspiration. Perspiration releases fluid through the pores of the skin.

Skin must effectively eliminate wastes from the body. The pores of the skin must be kept clean and open. The body must have an adequate supply of nutrients, to manufacture new, healthy cells for the skin. Healthy skin helps prevent microscopic parasites that breed and feed on wastes in the base of the hair follicle in the skin.

The skin takes in electrical energy from the air and sun. This energy is then absorbed through the skin into the bloodstream and assists in the making of red blood cells. These cells are produced mainly in the marrow of the bone. If the bone marrow is healthy and receiving essential oxygen, it will naturally produce more red blood cells as the body needs them.

► **THROUGH FOOD**

Fresh natural foods contain a form of pure distilled water and oxygen.

► **SIT UP STRAIGHT**

Sitting in a straight upright position allows the lungs to fill to full capacity.

► **TO INCREASE OXYGEN REFER TO ONE MINUTE EXERCISES (APPENDIX A)**

~ Chapter 4 ~

ASSIMILATION

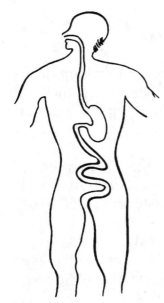

Everyone has different nutritional requirements. These requirements are based on eating habits, life style, work environment, and your present level of health.

A general description of *assimilation* is to take in, digest, and transform food into living tissue.

Digestion is a mechanical and chemical process. The mechanical process is carried out by the action of the muscles, and the chemical process by the action of the digestive fluids.

The *digestive tract* (the assimilation tract) consists of a tube approximately 30 feet long, from the mouth to the anus, lined by a mucous membrane. This tube is called the alimentary tract or canal, and consists of the mouth, esophagus, stomach, small intestines, and the large intestines.

DIGESTION

There are several essential principles of digestion that blend in with nature's process so subtly that mankind has overlooked them completely. Man is the highest form of creation, yet his digestive tract is designed for an *herbivorous diet*.

DISPLACED STOMACH

If the stomach is unable to begin breaking down the food because it is displaced or overloaded, the food begins to ferment, just as it would if you left it out on the table for too long.

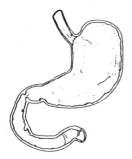

At this point, waste enters the blood-stream. The blood will deposit the waste anywhere in the body it can — the nose, ears, ovaries, prostate, lungs, liver, pancreas, gall bladder, or wherever there is a low resistance in the body.

VAGUS NERVE

If the stomach is displaced, it interferes with the very important vagus nerve which extends throughout the body. It is the vagus nerve that largely controls the production of *hydrochloric acid*, which is vital in digesting our foods.

THE STOMACH

In one way the stomach is very delicate. It can be pushed too far to the right or to the left. The top portion can be pushed or pulled up through the diaphragm (or breathing muscle). It may move up for only a few minutes or a few hours, and then drop back into place, so the symptoms you had for a while disappear. This symptom is sometimes referred to as the *hiatal hernia* (hiatal meaning "hole in the diaphragm", and hernia meaning "weakened or stretched").

STRESS

Stress can cause the top of stomach to ascend through the diaphragm. The stomach area is especially sensitive because it is the area of the solar plexus (between the rib cage) — one of the major nerve centers of the body.

Anger, fear, frustration, jealously, etc., may lead to many biochemical changes that produce excess acid in the body creating tension in the stomach.

We become sick when the body is *too acid*. The entire digestive process becomes affected when the acid-alkaline balance is upset.

A person can suffer from malnourishment even though he or she is getting plenty of food. (See section on Digestion.)

CONFUSING SYMPTOMS

When you have confusing symptoms of distress, the stomach or other digestive organs are generally the major cause. In many cases, the hiatal hernia is part of the problem. *If the stomach is raised, it does not digest and assimilate food well enough.* (Please refer to One- Minute Exercise.)

UNDIGESTED FOOD

The by-products of *undigested* food sometimes cause blockage, constipation and *fermentation of food in the intestines,* as well as lack of nutrition. *Cancer* cells proliferate and *multiply* in an environment of fermentation.

POOR DIGESTION

Poor digestion causes poor elimination. Other digestive difficulties caused by the hiatal hernia or displaced stomach are belching, bloating, intestinal gas, regurgitation (vomit), hiccups, nausea, constipation, and sometimes diarrhea. Symptoms change as the position of the stomach shifts.

DEEP BREATHING

In addition to digestive disorders, the displaced or ascended stomach interferes with deep breathing and circulation. When the stomach is ascended (pulled up) and pressed against the diaphragm (the breathing muscle of the lungs), reduced oxygen intake occurs. Dizziness can occur from *lack of oxygen* to the brain.

ORGANS

Every organ has its dwelling place in the body. Its function and dysfunction is coordinated with other organs. One organ out of place can cause problems with the other organs. Not only can the stomach get pulled up into the diaphragm, the lower part can get stretched out of shape by eating too much at a given time causing extra weight pushing against the sphincter ring (holding ring). This causes the food to pass through undigested along with acid that should remain in the stomach, sometimes causing *duodenum ulcers.*

THE FIRST PRINCIPLE: *chewing of starches.*

Chewing properly mixes the saliva with starch molecules. Saliva contains the enzyme ptyalin, which starts the digest process IN THE MOUTH. Digestion begins with the breaking up of fibrous envelopes or coverings of grasses and grains by means of mastication (chewing) and insalivation.

Starchy food should be chewed well in order to thoroughly mix it with saliva and thus the *enzyme ptyalin*, which acts upon the starches and prepares them for further digestion in the intestines. This is necessary because the principle digestion of starch STARTS IN THE MOUTH and finishes in the small intestines. That is why grass and grain eating animals (herbivores) spend so much time chewing their food. They grind it up thoroughly, mixing it with plenty of saliva to aid in digestion. This allows them to remain healthy, provided the food is suitable, and supplies all of the elements necessary for the life process.

In the human diet these simple facts have been totally overlooked in regard to the principles of digestive enzyme function and the <u>practice of chewing</u>. Because man doesn't make adequate time for this important part of the digestive process, he spends months in the hospital trying to patch up the damage this disregard of nature's law brings upon his body.

Dry prepared breakfast foods are usually drenched with hot or cold milk, cream, syrup, and/or sugar. This saturation leaves no room for the saliva to make direct contact with the starch molecules that need to be broken up by the saliva in order for proper digestion to take place.

The sad part of it is that this well-established breakfast habit, supposedly considered healthy, has caused many ills to the human race. This is hard to believe, until you trace it to the thousands of cases of indigestion and the trail of illness that follows. The after effect of this type of breakfast has been a big headache to many physicians and patients alike. *DIABETES* is <u>only one</u> of the many consequences of the body chemistry's *inability to assimilate* through the digestive system these unprocessed starches. The addition of white sugar and artificial sweeteners (*TAKEN DAILY*) also further inhibits this process.

In children, breakfasts like those mentioned above have caused a wide variety of catarrhal and mucous symptoms of the throat, nose, and sinuses, as well as tonsillitis, adenoids, eye and ear trouble, susceptibility to colds, and so forth.

Quoting from the late and great Dr. Randolph Stone, D.O., D.N., founder of the *polarity* therapy which I now practice and teach, — "For over 50 years I have searched for an answer to this problem in a busy practice. Until I found that even *ADULT INDIGESTION* is rarely diagnosed, properly treated, or relieved in general practices all over the world. This comes as a shock to me, particularly since I have been consulted by patients of wealth and means who have traveled to a dozen or more countries in an official capacity and also sought an answer to their health problems from eminent practitioners in these countries, but have found no relief. By the grace of God I was able to help them when all other methods have failed."

We can easily brush this off saying that the habits of the general public cannot be wrong, but they suffer just the same. (The proof being the widespread increase in the use of antacids, anti-flatulents, and digestive aids.) What needless suffering, when the cause can be pinpointed and solved!

There are many sick people who get well when they start *FLETCHERIZING* (chewing) their food, and as a result *EAT LESS*. Dr. Fletcher discovered this simple fact many years ago while he was very ill, and the proof was a healthy life after that. The name *fletcherizing* was given to this process of thorough and lengthy insalivation (the act of thoroughly mixing food with saliva). His book on fletcherizing is well known. The movement of the mouth releases saliva. A baby has milk only for the first six months or so. The *nursing action* releases the saliva to digest the milk.

Rice is a starch and when cooked properly, as it is in the Orient so that every kernel is whole and dry, it is the well established diet of millions. Poor people enjoy it, chew it well and stay well even when they have so little of it. This, of course, applies to the natural unprocessed, unpolished rice for which the value of the rice bran has not been removed.

Plain potatoes, boiled with the skins on, serve a similar purpose. Dr. Stone states, "This was the main diet of the peasantry in early Pomerania and Germany. They ate these potatoes only with sour skim milk (curd), and did not know what illness was with this simple mono diet, which included whole dark grain and bread without butter or ghee. They performed hard physical labor and so this diet was suited to their circumstances. But for the sedentary worker, potatoes may be a bit too heavy." He further asserts, "The simple diet and one suited to the *INDIVIDUAL NEED* is the one essential for health."

Dr. Metchnikoff called the world's attention to the Bulgarian peasants' diet of yogurt and acidophilus years ago. But when they consumed this with rich foods, fermentation and an acid reaction were caused in the system. Yogurt and acidophilus booths were quite a fad in the French Riviera some years ago, but the fad ceased when rheumatism set in due to this fermentation.

Excess amounts of *lactic acid* are one cause of sore joints and muscles. Illness resulted when people over-consumed the yogurt and acidophilus. In order to be beneficial, the yogurt and acidophilus should be taken in small quantities and *ONLY WHEN FRESH*.

THE SECOND PRINCIPLE: *protein foods need hydrochloric acid to digest in the stomach.*

That is why protein foods should be eaten first when they are part of a meal. This enables the protein of the meat, beans, lentils, peas, cheese, and so forth, to be coated by the juices in the stomach and become saturated with them before all other foods or drinks dilute the enzyme mixture of the hydrochloric acid in the stomach. That is why it is a good policy not to drink more than 2 to 4 ounces of liquid with meals, especially *NOT COLD DRINKS*, as they lower the temperature at which digestion takes place in the stomach. Rich protein foods with fats in them can cause real upset when a cold drink is taken with the meal. Cold drinks consumed with any animal protein can reduce the heat (sometimes the stomach heats to 105 degrees).

Fried foods are almost indigestible because food and oil become welded together at high cooking temperatures. These foods can become injurious to the liver and kidneys, and often produce liver symptoms and yellow jaundice. Also, cooking food in the usual way by adding oils and butter to the food during the cooking process does similar damage, but of a lesser degree. The body requires some oils. Why cook fats into foods at all? Why not add them when serving the food so that the high temperature of cooking won't weld them together, making them indigestible. Do the same with them as you would when adding oil and lemon to salads as a dressing. Most raw nuts contain oil.

THE THIRD PRINCIPLE: *only foods that are properly digested are useful in the body for its chemistry of replacing worn out tissue cells, minerals, vitamins, and enzymes.*

Fresh and natural foods receive their value from sunlight; which produces chlorophyll in *LEAVES, FRUITS, AND GRASSES*. These are the greatest nourishment to man and beast. A selection of these varieties give us *VITAL ENERGY REPLACEMENTS*. Plus, these vitamins, minerals, and concentrated proteins are lacking in over-cooked foods, as well as in chemically prepared substitutes and supplements.

The hidden or constant hunger is not caused by lack of food or lack of protein, but by a *LACK OF PROPER NUTRITION* and/or assimilation.

THE BREAKFAST PROBLEM

If you are not engaging in physically active labor, a heavy breakfast in the morning is a big mistake in the economy of the body's chemistry because all of the tubes and their mucus linings have been in a state of rest and repair during sleep. There is an exchange of secretions in their cellular tissues while in the relaxed state, so that they need *FLUSHING OUT IN THE MORNING* (the same as we would wash out our mouth, brush our teeth with cleansers or wash the tongue with a wash rag, giving us a refreshing, clean feeling). Some herb teas are recommended, as well as lemon, lime, or apple cider vinegar in the water. These are a great service and do an excellent job of flushing tissue cells.

Eating fruit 20 to 30 minutes before breakfast will assist in the exit of food from the stomach and assist in *digestion and elimination.*

Also recommended are fruit juices (*ALWAYS CONSUMED WHILE FRESH*), hot water and honey, and fresh vegetable juices from carrots or edible greens, celery, parsley, ginger root, zucchini or any vegetable in season. Most vegetable juices combine together well. Fruit juices, acid and sub-acid, will go fairly well together, as will sub-acid and sweet. Acid and sweet fruits do not combine together well. (Refer to Chapter 7, Foods Acid & Alkaline Balance.)

Melons, whether eaten or juiced, are best to eat or drink *alone*, or leave them alone.

Here it seems well worth repeating that only the foods that are properly digested and distributed in the body are useful in health building.

Carburization in a motor, and its oxidation of fuel, is a similar method to the digestive process in the body. *Carbonization or congestion is due to indigestion*, with its many hidden symptoms and ills. Stagnation in the digestive system promotes fermentation and breeds harmful bacteria.

MAKE YOUR TUMMY HAPPY

The moods we are in when partaking of food or drink have a great bearing on our digestive system. The best food may be indigestible if taken when one is in a state of anger, tension, or too much excitement. At such times it is advisable to partake of warm liquids only, thereby relaxing the stomach. Of course, the best remedy is to avoid such states in the first place, but if and when this does happen we only add insult to injury by loading the stomach with a heavy meal.

~ Chapter 5 ~

ENZYMES

Enzyme function is necessary for our breathing, growth, digestion, hormone action, blood coagulation, detoxification, perception of the senses, and reproduction. Every chemical action in the body depends on enzymes. All of our organs, glands, tissues, and cells are run by metabolic enzymes. Vitamins, minerals, and hormones need enzymes to do their work properly. Enzymes also represent the electrical energy for life force. We are wireless electricity.

The word enzyme comes from the Greek word meaning "leavened". *Enzyme* is a name given to substances that occur naturally in all living things, including the human body. ALL LIFE PROCESSES INVOLVE A SERIES OF CHEMICAL REACTIONS CALLED METABOLISM. **Metabolism sets enzymes in motion.** *Metabolism* is the name given to the chemical changes continually going on in the cells much like leaven in bread. Enzymes are the catalysts that makes metabolism possible.

ENZYME RESERVE

We are all born with a limited enzyme reserve. The quality of this reserve is decreased when our diet is deficient in enzymes.

Foods in their natural state are "live" foods (i.e., any fruits, nuts or vegetables grown from the earth), God-made, and still raw. *Live foods have their own enzyme supply.*

"Dead" foods are a "non-food" which are overcooked, processed, re-fortified, and refined foods that have been depleted of their naturally occurring enzymes and nutrients. Also, *fresh foods that have been picked too long, become a "non-food".*

We do not get energy from the food we eat; we get energy from the energy in the food we eat.

By eating mostly overcooked and processed foods, depleted of their naturally occurring enzymes, our digestive systems have to provide almost all of the enzymes needed for digestion, particularly when eating so-called dead foods.

The body draws on its enzyme reserves from all organs and tissues, causing *metabolic deficit* (the physical and chemical process that living things carry on to maintain life). This can cause an enlargement of the digestive organs and can lead to a variety of disorders and disease.

CATEGORIES OF FOOD ENZYMES

There are five categories of food enzymes, each having a specific function:
1. Lipase – Fats / Trypsin
2. Protease – Proteins / Pepsin

3.   Cellulase – Cellulose
4.   Amylase – Starch
5.   Rennin – Milk (lactose)

MAJOR GROUPS

Enzymes are also classified into two major groups:

1.   Exogenous – As in raw foods or supplements, enzymes taken in from the outside; and

2.   Endogenous – Enzymes produced within our bodies.

IMMUNE SYSTEM

It is important to have a good enzyme reserve for a healthy immune system. *Enzymes act as scavengers.* They latch on to foreign substances and reduce them so the body can rid itself of them.

TIPS TO GET FULL USE OF YOUR ENZYMES

▶   It is wise to consume your food at mealtimes (the sizable portion), whether it is 3 to 6 times a day as opposed to continually snacking a few bites throughout the day. Since every person has limited enzyme reserves, we can conserve our supply by eating mainly raw food snacks between meals.

▶ *The habit of drinking more than 4 ounces of any liquid at a meal should not be encouraged, since the liquids dilute the digestive fluids.* A warm temperature in the stomach is required for digestion to effectively take place. Cold liquids prevent the digestive action from promptly and properly working.

▶ Drinking water and beverages between meals is a must for proper elimination.

▶ Continually sipping water <u>stresses the kidneys</u>. Drink a substantial amount of water at one time, rather than a little sip now and then.

▶ If the stomach is over-extended with too much food at one time, it causes stress on the enzymes and depletes the reserve.

▶ Note that when you start eating, the food tastes good. The taste may change as the body says that is all of that particular kind of food that is needed at the time.

RAW FOOD

Enzymes from most raw food digest without the help of enzymes within the organs. It has been noted that eating a large percentage of raw food or taking enzyme supplements can help take the stress off not only the pancreas, but the entire body. A ratio of 80% fresh raw food to 20% cooked will ensure a good enzyme intake. Foods that have been canned, processed, smoked, pickled, fried, or cooked at high temperatures contain little or no enzymes. Enzyme rich foods are: sun-ripened raw fruits and vegetables and their juices, raw and sprouted seeds and nuts, and fresh or dried herbs. Enzymes in the dormant state are found usually in dry seeds and can keep their activity for hundreds of years.

PROTEINS

Eating too much flesh protein causes a decrease in enzyme, vitamin, and mineral levels. It is a good idea to have some raw vegetables with animal proteins, as the vegetables will supply the enzymes that are essential to the utilization of proteins.

HEALTH BENEFITS OF ENZYMES

A relaxed attitude before and after eating a meal lessens the need for so many enzymes. Tension causes *acidity*, causing the digestive organs to work harder.

Enzymes are a measure of vitality. The process of building up and breaking down all body tissues is done by enzymes. When the enzyme level is lowered, our metabolism is lowered, and as a result, so is our energy level. Any increase in *metabolic* activity — fevers, exercise, digestion, muscular work, or pregnancy — *uses up enzymes.*

People get tired when they are lacking in enzymes and

therefore the food they eat cannot be digested and utilized properly. The undigested food becomes waste matter and turns to toxins and poisons. It is estimated that approximately 80% of all disease is caused by toxins from improperly digested foods. Undigested molecules get absorbed into the bloodstream, and cause allergies or sickness.

ENZYMES ASSIST VITAMINS AND MINERALS

When combined with enzymes, smaller amounts of vitamins and minerals are needed because more of the nutrients are assimilated. Unless substances ingested contain their own enzymes, the body has to steal enzymes from all parts of itself, which lowers energy and causes aging. Supplemental enzymes taken with vitamins or food can help to offset this.

ENZYMES ARE NECESSARY FOR GLANDS AND HORMONES

The glands take up enzymes from raw foods and use them for metabolism, building billions of body tissues and cells, purifying the bloodstream, assimilating nutrients, and nourishing all the body organs.

Enzymes are sometimes called "hormone youth factories". Hormones use the fiber of raw foods to give the digestive organs an internal scrubbing. Nutrients and enzymes from raw foods are used to enrich the quality of the bloodstream.

BLOOD USES ENZYMES

Our blood uses enzyme-enriched hormones to absorb oxygen in the lungs and carries it to every body part. Blood carries waste products from the various body tissues to the kidneys and other organs of elimination. Through this process, *enzymes offer the key to longevity,* and they seem to be able to neutralize the basic causes of *aging* in the body. The more we maintain our enzyme reserve, the healthier we will be. Of the more than *700 different enzymatic hormones in the system,* each one has its individual benefit. The absence or weakening of any enzyme slows down the entire glandular network.

When blood cannot circulate to the cells that make up this physical temple, or when the blood is toxic or un-oxygenated, the cells do not get fed or cleansed; thus they begin to die. When cells begin to die in some areas of the body, it is just a matter of time before symptoms are experienced.

~ 1 Corinthians 12:26 ~

"And whether one member suffer, all the members suffer with it; or one member be honoured, all the members rejoice with it."

~ Chapter 6 ~

ORGANS
THEIR LOCATION
AND FUNCTION

STOMACH

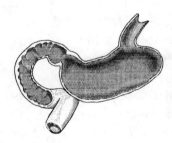

The stomach is a muscular pouch located on the left side of the upper part of the abdomen just under the lower tips of the rib cage. Its right side is overlapped by the liver. The outer surface of the stomach is smooth. The inner surface is folded into numerous complex ridges which assist in the mixing of food with digestive juices and channel this material through the stomach into the intestines. *Only water, alcohol, and certain drugs seem to be absorbed from the stomach.* Most food assimilation and absorption takes place in the small intestine.

The walls of the empty stomach are in contact with each other. As food enters the stomach, the walls yield and the stomach enlarges without change in intragastric pressure. The upper portion of the stomach stores the ingested food (food just eaten). Waves of contraction of the circular muscle, preceded by waves of relaxation (*peristalsis*), start about midway in the stomach and travel downward. Such waves of contractions, which may occur at a rate of three per minute, break up and thoroughly mix the food with gastric juice.

The innermost layer, *the mucosa*, contains secretory cells. One type secretes hydrochloric acid, which not only neutralizes the alkaline reaction of the saliva, but renders the gastric contents distinctly acid and activates the gastric digestive juices. These juices are secreted by a different type of cell. The enzymes found in gastric juices are pepsin, which in the presence of acid splits proteins to peptones; rennin, which curdles milk; and perhaps lipase, which splits fats to fatty acids and glycerol. A third type of cell secretes mucus for the protection of the stomach from its own products.

Meat, cooked grains, and partly digested products of proteins stimulate the flow of gastric juices. Gastric secretion also may be stimulated by the mere sight or smell of food.

Discharging of food from the stomach into the *duodenum* (the first 8 inches of the small intestine) is caused by the contraction of the muscles in the stomach wall. These muscles are innervated by the cranial vagus nerves, which stimulate contraction of the gastric musculature and allow the sphincter (holding ring) between the stomach and the duodenum to open. The stomach, like the heart, must be regarded as an automatic organ. Whether the automaticity is determined in the musculature or in an intrinsic nerve mechanism is unknown. Sympathetic nerve fibers in the splanchnic nerves have opposite effects to the vagal nerves, preventing gastric emptying.

LIVER - GALL BLADDER

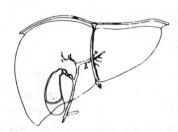

The liver is the principal detoxifying organ of the body. It performs the miracle of converting our food into living energy. It acts as a blood reservoir. Approximately one-fourth of the blood in a healthy body is in the liver at all times. Blood comes to the liver, stomach, spleen, pancreas, and intestines through the oxygenation process.

The liver filters out waste and other poisons, filtering more than a quart a minute. The liver produces bile which assists digestion. Bile is a yellow or black fluid which is as bitter as gall (gall being another name for it).

The liver rebuilds, repairs, rejuvenates and regenerates. This is called the "4 R's" of the liver.

In ancient times, the liver and gall bladder were associated with human emotions and dispositions called the 4 humors: blood, phlegm, black and yellow bile, reflected in the words choleric, melancholy, bilious, jaundice, and liverish. "Chol" means bile or gall. According to the dictionary, in 1653, over three hundred years ago, melancholy literally means "black bile", one of the most depressing kinds. A person affected by the humor could have symptoms of being depressed and scared, gloomy, dejected, sullen, dismal or sad.

The antidote for changing the chemical in the liver was laughter and still applies today.

Proverbs 17:22 – *"A merry heart doeth good like a medicine; but a broken spirit drieth the bones."*

The gallbladder is a storage organ which concentrates the bile approximately ten times. It has a muscle layer which contracts at appropriate times and squeezes alkaline bile into the duodenum (the upper part of the small intestine).

A high acid meal particularly needs the powerful concentrations of bile to alkalize the intestine. The very sight, thought, or taste of food is sufficient to start the emptying of the gallbladder. When the gall bladder empties prematurely, it can cause extra stress on the liver, as the liver has to work harder to produce more bile.

This is one reason chewing gum causes stress on the body — *except right after eating.* The taste of the chewing gum causes the gall bladder to begin to dump the bile, and the body begins to secrete enzymes to digest the gum. Then spit is produced and you swallow. You then need a different enzyme to digest the saliva. Saliva is alkaline. Chewing gum is acid. The stomach is prepared to digest the gum. This uses up precious enzymes of the body and stresses the liver at the same time. Most people do not realize how hard the body has to work when they chew gum.

The best time to chew gum would be just after eating while the digestive system is still working, or very briefly as a breath freshener.

SMALL INTESTINE

The small intestine is where major assimilation takes place. It is a coiled tube about 23 feet long of four coats. For identification it is divided into three portions: the *duodenum, the jejunum and the ileum.* The upper part beginning at the bottom opening of the stomach is the duodenum and is about 8 inches long. The ducts from the liver and pancreas open into this part of the intestines about 6 inches from the stomach. The jejunum continues from the duodenum and is about 7.5 feet long, and lies mostly in the umbilical (belly button) region and left iliac. The *ileum* (bottom of left rib cage) forms the remainder of the small intestine and connects near the right hip bone with the colon (the large gut). The opening from the ileum into the colon is the ileo-cecal valve, which allows no regurgitation or reentering of the processed food back into the small intestine.

When the food arrives into the small intestines, it is further acted upon by the intestinal, pancreatic, and biliary juices which are of an alkaline medium.

The mucous membrane of the small intestine contains a massive number of small finger-like projections called villi and each villus has a lymphatic called a lacteal. When the digested food becomes a milk-like fluid, it is ready for absorption. This fluid is called chyme. Digested fat from the intestine passes into the lacteals and then into the lymphatics which empty into the thoracic duct and from there into the subclavian vein. The digested protein and carbohydrates are collected by the venous (blood) capillaries of the portal system and carried to the liver. The undigested material passes into the colon and is known as the feces or fecal matter.

ADRENALS

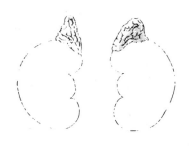

The pair of adrenal glands are located on top of the kidneys. The adrenals are ductless glands that are responsible for producing some of the most important hormones in the body. All glands of the body are classified as either endocrine (secreting internally rather than through a duct) or exocrine (having a secretion through a duct). The secretions of endocrine glands are always hormones that regulate various activities and functions.

The production of important adrenal hormones always requires active work by the cells and results in exchange of energy. The harmonizing balance in the body requires that a proper amount of nutrients be available in the blood to allow for the quick response to an increase in energy needs.

PANCREAS

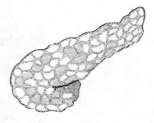

The pancreas is a soft, reddish or yellowish gland which lies behind the stomach. It is about 5 inches long and about 2 inches wide. The right end of the pancreas is attached to the duodenum (the first 8 inches of the small intestines), and the left end is attached to the spleen.

The pancreas has both an exocrine and an endocrine secretion. The exocrine secretion is made up of a number of enzymes that are discharged into the intestine to aid in digestion. The endocrine secretion, insulin, is important in the metabolism of sugar in the body. Insulin is produced in small groups of especially modified glandular cells in the pancreas; these cell groups are known as the islets of Langerhans. The failure of these cells to secrete sufficient amounts of insulin causes diabetes.

The pancreas is a multi-faceted organ and plays a major role in digesting our food. It will take sugar and starch from our food and turn them into heat and energy. Disregarding the balanced intake of sugar and starch can make the pancreas over- or under-active.

THYROID

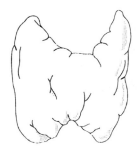

The *thyroid gland* is located in the neck. It is made up of two lobes connected in the middle by a mass of tissue. The thyroid gland is slightly larger in women than in men. The functions of the thyroid's hormones are threefold: (1) cellular metabolism, (2) growth and development, and (3) oxygen use. The thyroid gland releases the hormone thyroxin directly into the blood. The hormone calcitonin is essential. It influences calcium homeostasis. These two hormones require a trace mineral called iodine.

PROSTATE

The *prostate gland* is the largest gland of the male reproductive tract. It is located directly under the urinary bladder. The prostate is similar in size and texture to a chestnut. It is placed in the pelvic cavity and rests about 1.5 inches inside the rectum. The prostate may be distinctly felt upon examination, especially when enlarged.

The function of the prostate is to secrete a milky, slightly acidic fluid into the *prostatic urethra*. The urethra is the terminal canal for the male reproductive and urinary systems and serves as a passageway for the different fluids to form semen, the male reproductive fluid. Prostatic fluid contains enzymes which balance the acid level.

There is a good deal of research being conducted on the prostate, yet it remains one of the least understood structures in the body.

The beginning of a problem could occur when the penis is pressed against the wall of the woman's uterus, restricting the flow of semen during normal ejaculation. This continued practice could weaken the sphincter ring that holds the blood in the penis during intercourse. The same problem could occur during masturbation if the penis is held too tight during ejaculation.

Should you remain celibate, total abstinence from sexual activity, this does not apply to you.

Sex is the number one exercise to enable the prostate to keep a fresh supply of oxygenated blood exchanged. The major time the prostate should become hard is from the beginning to the peak of a climax, not so much through thought or foreplay. The pulsation of the climax pumps the excess fluids, returning the prostate to its safe, flexible state.

THE BODY'S SECURITY SYSTEM

Food
Acid And Alkaline
Balance

~ Chapter 7 ~

FOOD
ACID AND ALKALINE
BALANCE

It is not the actual acid-alkaline measurement of food itself that is influencing our health, but rather the acidity or alkalinity of the ash or residue that is formed. Some foods such as lemons and limes contain strong acid, but the condition they cause in the body after digestion is alkaline.

A RESIDUE CALLED ASH

During the digestion process food is combined with oxygen, using and producing energy in the body. After the nutrients have been absorbed and utilized, the result is a residue called ash which is left in the digestive tract. This residue becomes fecal matter. This is similar to the ashes left from the burning of wood.

Acid foods are primarily proteins and starches. *Alkaline foods* are mostly fruits and vegetables. A chart reflecting how the food reacts in the body, rather than a chemical analysis of the food itself.

ACID-ALKALINE FOOD CHARTS
FOODS THAT FORM ACID ASH

1. Alcohol
2. Beans (dried, except lima and azuki)
3. Bananas (if green tipped)
4. Bread
5. Caffeine
6. Cereals
7. Coffee
8. Cheese (all kinds)
9. Chocolate
10. Coconuts (dried)
11. Cranberries
12. Flour and grains (wheat, rye, oats, millet, buckwheat, soy)
13. Lentils
14. Meat (including fowl, fish, and shellfish)
15. Milk (pasteurized and homogenized products)
16. Nuts (except almonds and chestnuts)
17. Oranges and juice
18. Pasta (all forms)
19. Peanuts
20. Pineapple
21. Seeds (unless sprouted)
22. Strawberries
23. Sugar
24. Tea (except herbal)
25. Tapioca

FOODS THAT FORM ALKALINE ASH

VEGETABLES AND HERBS

1. Agar
2. Alfalfa
3. Artichokes (all kinds)
4. Asparagus
5. Bamboo Shoots
6. Beans (azuki, green or string, limas - dry or fresh)
7. Bean Sprouts
8. Beets and Tops
9. Bok Choy
10. Broccoli
11. Burdock
12. Cabbage (red, white, Chinese)
13. Cauliflower
14. Carrot
15. Celery
16. Chicory
17. Chives
18. Cloves
19. Collards
20. Clowslip
21. Corn (fresh and sweet)
22. Cucumber
23. Daikon Radish
24. Dandelion
25. Dill
26. Dock
27. Dulse
28. Endive
30. Garlic
31. Ginger
32. Horseradish (fresh)
33. Horsetail
34. Kale
35. Kelp
36. Kohlrabi
37. Kombu, Limas (dry or fresh)
38. Leeks
39. Lettuce (all kinds)
40. Lotus Root
41. Mustard Greens
42. Olives
43. Okra
44. Onions
45. Parsley
46. Parsnip
47. Peas (green)
48. Pepper (green, yellow, red)
49. Potatoes (with peeling)
50. Prickly Pear
51. Radish
52. Sage
53. Sauerkraut (brines)
54. Sorrel
55. Soybeans and Soybean Extract

56. Spinach
57. Sprouts
58. Squash (all kinds)
59. Swiss Chard
60. Turnips and Tops
61. Water Chestnuts
62. Watercress
63. Zucchini

FRUITS

1. Apples and Apple Cider
2. Apricots
3. Banana (speckled only)
4. Blackberries
5. Boysenberries
6. Cherries
7. Currants
8. Dates
9. Figs
10. Grapefruit
11. Grapes
12. Lemons & Peel
13. Limes
14. Loganberries
15. Mango
16. Melons (all kinds)
17. Papaya
18. Passion Fruit
19. Peach
20. Pear
21. Plums
22. Persimmons
23. Pomegranate
24. Prunes
25. Raisins

MISCELLANEOUS

1. Acidophilus
2. Coconut (fresh)
3. Honey
4. Miso
5. Molasses
6. Mushrooms (raw - most varieties)
7. Pure Apple Cider Vinegar

8. Sprouted Seeds
9. Teas (herbal, unsweetened)

DAIRY

1. Buttermilk
2. Milk (raw)
3. Whey
4. Yogurt (homemade used within 48 hours)

NEUTRAL

1. Avocado
2. Butter
3. Oils

NEUTRALIZING EXCESS ACID

Every *acid*-forming food leaves an acid residue behind that must be neutralized to prevent chemical imbalance in the cells.

The *alkaline* foods create valuable minerals including magnesium, calcium, potassium, and sodium, which the body uses to neutralize excess acids, thus preventing tissue damage.

Because the average American diet is predominantly acid, and fewer alkaline foods are eaten, our alkaline mineral reserve is low or depleted. Therefore there is an overabundance of acids that must be neutralized.

The average diet does not provide enough fruits

and vegetables to supply the materials needed for our alkaline reserve. This situation leads to acid cells. When enough cells reach this stage, the organ in which they reside becomes susceptible to infection, malfunction or chronic degeneration.

It is important to keep a good balance. It has been estimated that *the body needs approximately 80% alkaline foods and 20% acid foods.* When our diet contains this balance, we are getting a good building foundation to rejuvenate and regenerate our bodies and maintain a healthy lifestyle.

Excess animal protein depletes the body of energy because it uses more energy for digestion than it produces. Therefore, too much nitrogen is produced, causing fatigue. The residue left after eating meat becomes acid ash in the bloodstream, which has to be neutralized by the body's store of alkaline ash. When this reserve runs out, the body becomes acidic. Calcium is drawn from the bones as a neutralizing agent, resulting in a weakening of the bones. The immune system is then thrown out of balance, leaving the body susceptible to disease.

Live enzymes from fresh fruits and vegetables supply the alkaline ash or good chemical balance.

STANDARD AMERICAN DIET

All meat (flesh) – beef, pork, fish, fowl, and all processed foods are acid. These foods *taken in overabundance* deprives the nerves and the brain of needed oxygen, making us nervous, irritable, aggressive, in a negative, ill-tempered.

For example: The meat-eating animals, lion, tigers, etc., are aggressive, easily irritated, easily provoked. Grass and grain "vegetable" eating animals, regardless of their size, are of a calmer nature.

An individual consuming our standard American diet, regardless they are an adult, teenage or child, can become noticeably irritable, tired, or unusually aggressive when consuming excessive amounts of meat, imitation meat, as well as devitalized food.

STRESS AND NEGATIVE EMOTIONS CAUSE ACID

The more stress we accumulate in our body, whether emotional or physical, the more *acid* our entire system becomes.

Rest and sleep are alkalinizers, as well as fresh air, laughter, and expressions of love and well-being.

Negative emotions such as fear, worry, anger, envy, and greed are acidifiers. The emotions affect the body through the glandular system. Glands feed upon body secretions. When these secretions become poisoned by our negative thoughts, actions and feelings, our glands have to work overtime to eliminate the acidic toxins.

The high water content of fruits and vegetables help to hydrate the body, which aids our system in the ability to cast off the poisonous waste products of the tissues and cells.

PH SCALE

The chemical term for the relative acidity/ alkalinity is referred to as PH. The PH scale is from 1 to 14, with 7 representing neutrality — neither acid or alkaline. Most living things require an acid-alkaline environment between PH 5.5 and 8 to survive. The normal PH for human blood plasma is from 7.35 to 7.45, which is slightly alkaline. This is also the optimum range for human tissue. Certain organs in the body maintain a higher acidity than other organs and tissues. The body works hard to maintain this type of chemical balance.

Our bodies are in a state of constant change. The raw materials of our daily diet influence whether we are changing toward rejuvenation or degeneration.

BREAKING A HABIT

by John Boyle O'Reilly

How shall I a habit break?
As you did that habit make.
As you yielded, now refuse.
Thread by thread the strands we twist,
Till they bind us, neck and wrist.
Thread by thread, the patient hand,
Must untwine, ere free we stand.

~ Chapter 8~

ELIMINATION

Elimination and assimilation are two basic needs for natural health, and work hand in hand. If the *elimination organs* (the bowel, the kidneys, the skin and the lungs) are not functioning perfectly the body soon becomes choked with putrefying garbage backing up into all the vital organs. Assimilation then will be stifled and the end result will be death.

LARGE INTESTINE

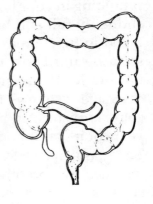

The large intestine or colon is about 5 to 6 feet in length and runs from the small intestine to the anus where it ends. The entrance of the colon is known as the cecum which is about 2.5 inches long. From the lower end of the cecum protrudes a small worm-like tube from 3 to 5 inches long called the appendix (vermiform appendix).

The *colon* is divided into *three parts* called the *ascending, transverse,* and *descending.* The ascending colon extends from the cecum up to the right side to the under surface of the liver. From there it makes a turn, called the *hepatic flexure* and runs across the upper abdomen below the liver and stomach to the spleen on the left side. This is known as the *transverse* colon. From the spleen it makes a turn called the *spleenic flexure* and runs downward to the hip bone and is known as the *descending* colon. At the top of the pelvis it makes an s-shaped curve called the *Sigmoid flexure*. From the Sigmoid flexure the colon is known as the *rectum* and terminates at the *anus*. The *anus* is surrounded by the external and internal sphincter muscles. These muscles close the exit of the bowels.

The colon functions for the most part as a kind of septic tank into which all of the filter organs, chiefly the liver, release their loads of accumulated toxic wastes which they have gathered from every part of the body through the blood and lymph systems. Can you imagine the plumbing in your home if the septic tank or sewer were suddenly full and backing up? Or even if the system failed to function as required? The house would very soon be unfit for habitation. Your organs — liver, gallbladder, pancreas, spleen, kidneys and your drainage system — function like plumbing. When the colon is obstructed by accumulated wastes (sometimes years of it), your body is faced with a similar situation. The maintenance system breaks down. The liver, for instance, has no other recourse than to reluctantly *recycle wastes back into your tissues.* This unhealthy occurrence is epidemic in America, and has been termed <u>intestinal toxemia</u> or <u>auto-intoxication</u>. It means you can be poisoning yourself in your own undischarged wastes.

We become careless of responding to the "calls of nature" to empty the bowel, because we have thought of the lower bowel as a sort of reservoir for the non-digestible and non-absorbable food waste, wherein it may be held until it suits the convenience or the whim of the individual to discharge. *When we resist the call, the peristaltic action that brought the feces to the rectum to be evacuated reverses and carries the feces (stool) further up into the colon.*

In most people this is a slow process in which the various waste toxins (plaque), build up over a period of years to produce arthritis, ulcers, cancer, diabetes, hypertension, heart attacks, strokes, etc. Many patients experience only headaches or a sluggish tired feeling as warning symptoms for months or years before the final breakdown.

Before the advent of devitalized foods and water, coupled with sedentary living, elimination was not the problem it is today. A "normal" colon is found today in very few people. Instead, most people today feeding on non-foods along with excess stress, have colons replete with abnormal pockets, bulges, twists, and crooks. These can harbor impacted cement-like waste deposits adhering to the colon walls, and often serve as home for various parasites and harmful bacteria.

You may be constipated even while having bowel movements two or three times daily. But let us consider for a moment the concept of real natural elimination which should be part of your natural health heritage. You were designed by our Creator to have a complete evacuation of the lower bowel at least one time daily when eating a substantial meal. A complete evacuation is not to be confused with small partial eliminations which most people experience, nor can the partial give the same feeling of freedom, energy and vibrant well-being.

The bowel is our friend. It is working 24 hours a day to rid the body of toxins and plaque build-up. Remove the plaque or it will remove you!

Now it may surprise you to learn that evacuating while sitting on a toilet is about as natural as eating while standing on your head. You were designed to evacuate in a natural squatting position with your weight on your feet. This is nature's way of promoting the peristaltic action necessary for complete evacuation. Any other way impedes nature's purpose.

In my opinion, *all sicknesses are related to elimination problems* — either directly or indirectly. The word "physician" comes from the word "physic" of which one of the meanings is laxative.

Putrefaction makes the colon become stagnant and weak. Germs live in any kind of waste which the body cannot assimilate, utilize or eliminate. It is of vital importance to get rid of waste matter before it gets stored in the tissues. Food should be eliminated within 18 to 22 hours. Otherwise, pests and bacteria begin breeding.

Matthew 15:17 — *"Perceive ye not that whatsoever goeth into the mouth passeth into the belly and is cast out into the draught."*

PARASITES

A parasite is anything that lives off of something else. Approximately 80% of the population has worms, some of which can be seen only with a microscope. Parasites set up colonies in the *bowel*. Parasites can move into the bloodstream from the colon walls and be deposited into other tissues and organs of the body. If the immune system is low, they are able to stay in the body.

There are several places to look for parasites.

In the toilet - A parasite that has been showing up in colon therapy clients of mine for the past nine years is one that I refer to as the black hair worm. It might look like a cotton ball with dark thin hair-like lines similar to an eyelash. The ball can vary in size up to the width of a thumbnail. They can sometimes be detected in a bowel movement with careful observation.

In the nostril - I have discovered a different parasite in my own nostrils. They are white and flat, up to ½" long, and have elasticity. They look like a narrow flat piece of rubber band. They run horizontal with the nose and feel like a little ridge attached inside the nostril. They sometimes come out with the mucous and would not be detected unless very closely observed. I have also found this type of parasite in fish and chicken.

If we allow the bowel to remain stagnant by not giving it enough nutrition from fruits, vegetables, nuts and seeds, and pure water, it cannot be nourished, and waste matter builds upon the colon walls.

If your colon has never been cleared of the mucous and impacted waste that builds up over the years, it is almost impossible to achieve maximum health. *When the colon becomes clogged, it poisons the entire body.*

CONSTIPATION

Constipation seems far more of a universal complaint today than ever before judging by those of us who come into personal contact with the American public on a confidential basis. One of the first questions the old family doctor used to ask, was "How are your bowels?" Today this seems to be an old-fashioned and forgotten question with many doctors.

In times past, when you were sick, the doctor would in some way move your bowels and that was "health".

I remember my mom asking me to stick out my tongue. I did not know what she was looking for but hoped she did not find it, because I got either Castor Oil or Black Draught! She looked for a white or brownish coating on the tongue – "a coated tongue, a coated gut." (Please refer to One Minute Exercises to thoroughly cleanse the tongue as opposed to brushing with a toothbrush.)

Constipation is still a major health problem and should be more thoroughly understood by the individuals affected.

The most noticeable symptoms of a possible colon

problem are: chronic fatigue, irritability, facial skin blemishes, insomnia, foul-smelling gas, uncontrollable appetite, mental depression, offensive breath, menstrual pains, and a protruding abdomen. Your colon is intimately related to every part of your body. Few people realize how directly a malfunctioning colon is related to glandular disturbances, weariness, stress, and nervousness. So, if you feel your general health is lacking even though you are eating good food and taking proper mineral/vitamin supplements, you should give some attention to your digestion and colon health.

Why is colon health important? *The colon is the large intestine and the body's sewage system.* The indigestible portions of the food you eat lodge in the large intestine and stay there until eliminated in a bowel movement. Infrequent movements or periods of constipation can result in a partial decomposition of these waste substances that encrusts the colon and further hinders elimination, and allows toxins to build up in the colon. Since the skin is the largest organ of elimination, the body often attempts to eliminate these excess toxins through the skin. One key to healthy *skin* is having a *healthy efficient colon.*

AIDS TO PREVENT CONSTIPATION

Immediate attention to the call of nature is of the utmost importance. If the bowels are not allowed to evacuate at the appropriate time, the stool loses moisture and becomes hard and causes constipation.

Allow time for the urge to develop. Sometimes if one needs to urinate, and will allow extra time, the body will signal the bowels to evacuate also.

Eat fruit that contains its own juice, like peaches, pears, grapes, apples, etc. The apple contains pectin. The intestines contain pectin. So the apple feeds the colon. As the old saying states, "An apple a day keeps the doctor away."

Feces or fecal matter represents the residual food mass that remains in the large intestine after the full exercise of the digestive functions. Fecal matter is composed of the following substances:

1. Food residues:
    » Those portions of food which have escaped absorption.
    » That part of the diet either not digested or incapable of being absorbed.

2. The remains of the digestive and intestinal secretions not destroyed or reabsorbed.

3. The bacterial flora of the intestinal tract.

4. Cellular elements, which in pathological conditions may include blood, pub, mucus, serum, and parasites.

The amount of fecal discharge depends on the amount and kind of food ingested. *A heavy vegetable diet gives the greatest bowel movement.*

An enema is not the same as the colonic irrigation. It cleanses the lower bowel rather than the entire colon. It can be a valuable aid in getting the bowels to move when constipated, even if only a small amount of liquid is used.

THE COLEMA™ BOARD

The Colema™ Board (which is a type of enema kit) makes possible a program of colon cleansing when needed and desired. It is offered as a useful aid for keeping the colon clean. This is recommended by a company as a simple unit which can be used in the privacy of your own home. These five gallon colonics are vitally important to cleansing the colon properly. (See ordering information at the back of the book)

COLON IRRIGATION

Washing deteriorating waste from the intestines is the quickest way known to begin detoxification, the first step to natural health. The most immediate way to detoxify the colon is by colon irrigation, which can be done professionally or at home with the use of a Colema™ Board. There is more than one kind of professional colonic equipment. Most of the objection to colon irrigation comes from those who have experienced colonics from a pressurized machine, as opposed to the gentle gravity-flow machine.

Most of those reluctant to undergo colon irrigation and enemas are those who have had little or no experience with these gentle natural detoxifiers. Some say that colon irrigation washes out intestinal flora, valuable nutrients, and is habit forming. The truth is that the *washing out of putrefaction in the large intestine, which is the only part reached in any colon irrigation,* increases the good intestinal flora which can only breed in a clean environment which has been washed free of putrefaction and its accompanying harmful bacteria. That is why the intestines of a newborn baby immediately begin to grow good intestinal flora. Each time you clean out the putrefying garbage you make a better environment for the natural flora which start to multiply immediately in their natural media.

The intestines are muscles with nerves which normally trigger peristaltic contractions when the colon is full. Putrefaction makes the colon become stagnant and weak. But each time you fill the intestines with water, you cause these muscles and nerves to contract with new life. An arm or leg which is not exercised soon becomes flabby and weak. The same holds true for your colon. Yes, it is dependent upon both exercise and cleanliness. Colon irrigation is another way to supply both to correct unnatural conditions of filth and stagnation.

Sometimes a patient will feel nauseated and have some cramping during the intestinal wash. This is a certain indication that toxins are being released.

The intestinal wash can lower a high fever in minutes, much quicker than the most powerful antibiotic. Most headaches are rooted in intestinal putrefaction and often respond in minutes to a good intestinal wash.

Most patients are surprised at the fantastic results from the intestinal wash program they did not even think they needed. Improved digestion, increased mental power and sense of well-being, and more vibrant health are only a few of the benefits. We have seen patients with extreme depression and pessimism transformed into cheerful optimists after the putrefying waste was removed from their colon. And now you to can try it and see for yourself.

ELIMINATION THROUGH THE KIDNEYS

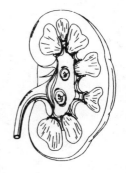

The body has two kidneys, each about 4-5 inches in length and reddish in color. The kidneys are located just above the waist, behind the abdominal cavity. The right kidney is slightly lower than the left, making room for the liver. In addition to their excretory function, the kidneys also *regulate body water* and the concentrations of essential electrolytes, such as sodium, potassium, calcium, phosphorus, chloride, bicarbonate, and many biologically valuable organic compounds, such as glucose and amino acids. They also help to regulate body pH by excreting acid.

Its basic functions include filtration, secretion, and reabsorption. It is obvious that several feedback systems are in place, working at maintaining proper acid/ alkaline balance. The normal kidney controls the excretion of electrolytes, water, and acid conveying the urine from the kidney to the outside. *The urinary system operates as a valuable tool to maintain the blood system.* It serves as the filter unit, adds nutrients back into the blood, and works to maintain the pH balance. The kidneys are responsible for the manufacturing of ammonia and glutamate. (Ammonia is the end product of protein metabolism.)

The kidneys work to nourish and clean the body and disposes of its pollution in a controlled and sensible manner.

~ Chapter 9 ~

JEANNIE'S QUOTES AND THOUGHTS PROVERBS OF HEALTH

▶ Healing is within our power. Miracles are within God's power.

▶ Harmful means different things to different people.

▶ A healthy body does *not* store excess fat.

▶ Inspiration is great. Information, when acted upon, is greater.

▶ Nutrition is a complete cycle.

▶ Joy is the best preventative medicine and balances the entire system.
   Q. How do I get joy?
   R. In His presence. (Psalms 16:1.)

STRESS: Is anything that interferes with smooth and easy operation of an object, an organism or a body. A bridge collapses, a rope breaks, people have ulcers, etc.

▶   Ancient proverb: to sleep is peace, to wake is joy.

▶   When negative emotions are strong, the bowel is stressed and shuts down, and the bile does not flow freely.

▶   The *best* food for balancing the bile are green tipped or leafy vegetables.

▶   Every thing that is alive has to be *fed*.

The creative mind has no limits. The conscious mind limits our subconscious.
   ▶   Positive: being able to visualize the results consciously.
   ▶   Negative: limiting oneself from taking action.
   ▶   Goals and dreams.

✳ ✳ ✳

Bowel: Feces that float is fiber (alkaline).
         Feces that sink is bulk (acid).
   Q.   How long should I eat fiber or high roughage?
   R.   As long as you want to feel good.

Estimated Needs:

Vegetables	60%
Fruits	20%
Starch	10%
Protein	10%

Consider protein and starch acid, fruits and vegetables alkaline.

* * *

Water: Drink regular tap water when no other is available.
▶ Drink water from hot water faucet.
▶ Drink before it is hot. May set aside to cool.
▶ The heating can help to purify the water.

One parasite I am finding seems to be water related.

* * *

Environment can contribute to our ills. Most of us prefer to believe that the illnesses we suffer are the results of external forces, bad luck or failure. We continue to say we "catch" a cold, "get" the flu and "contract" pneumonia, *as if we are in no way to blame for the medical catastrophes that befall us.*

* * *

I am convinced that every disease, physical and mental, is generated by a combination of circumstances which arise both inside and outside the body.

It logically follows that disease may be prevented or cured by correcting variables that exist both inside and outside the body. We can go after the cause, but we can also correct the life condition which predisposed the individual to illness. Such as: emotional illness, chemical deficiency, stresses, or interpersonal conflicts.

— • — • —

Should you have a birth defect or crippling disease, do the best you can to keep the body healthy through acid-alkaline balance.

— • — • —

BABY – Crying, crying, crying!!! Check mouth for ropy sticky saliva. If present, give a small quantity of water.

— • — • —

More and more babies today are being born with deficient immune systems and parasites already in their bodies. They are having bowel movements in the womb because their little bodies are already eliminating toxins that the mother has ingested. Should the baby's bowel move before birth, there is the possibility of the fluid surrounding the body becoming contaminated. When this occurs, they can nurse the fecal material back into their body. It has been known to cause serious illness or death. This can be avoided if the mother will take responsibility for her own body during pregnancy.

In summer animals eat green grasses and stay cool. In the winter they eat dry grasses and grains and stay warm. To stay cool in the summer, humans need to eat vegetables; to stay warm in the winter, eat grains and tubers. Fruits and vegetables are needed all year, as follows:

▶ Summer - fresh,
▶ Winter - more nuts, grains, fruit, squash, potatoes, onions, etc. (Food that does not require refrigeration.)

— • — • —

LEARN TO BELCH, IT COULD SAVE YOUR LIFE.

— • — • —

"Everybody needs a hug. It changes your metabolism." Philosopher Leo Buscaglia

— • — • —

It is my desire to share wisdom about how life is manifested within the physical body. We know we are indeed "fearfully and wonderfully made", according to Psalms 139:14. God created the body to operate within these physical laws. Once we understand these laws, we can see that the body is indeed "fearfully and wonderfully made" — not because of its complexity, but because of its simplicity.

— • — • —

MAY HEALTH FOREVER BE YOURS!

~ APPENDIX A ~

ONE MINUTE EXERCISES

HAIR

▶ With fingertips, begin at hairline running all ten fingers through your hair close to the scalp. Crush hair in the hands, grasping firmly with all fingers. Hold and release. Repeat ten to twelve times.

EYES

▶ Look up, look down, look left, look right.

▶ With eyelids closed, very gently press across the top of the closed eye with the tip of the thumb.

▶ With the tip of the middle finger, very gently press across under the eye.

EARS

▶ With fingers and thumb, massage entire ear inside and out, especially tender spots. Pull ear away from the head. This is a good stress release.

TONGUE

▶ With a dry wash cloth, start at the back of the tongue and pull forward toward the tip of the tongue. This will help remove the built up plaque on the tongue. You may then wet the wash cloth and wipe the tongue.

▶ Stick tongue out. Pull tongue in. Roll or fold, bringing outer sides of tongue together. Repeat ten or twelve times.

▶ A flexible tongue means a flexible body.

BREATHING

Breathing through the nostrils lead to health and well-being.

Breathing through the mouth leads to sickness and disease.

▶ With the right thumb on the right side of the nostril, blocking the airway, breathe air in through the left nostril and blow it out through the mouth. Repeat four to eight times.

▶ With the left thumb on the left side of the

nostril, blocking the airway, breathe air in through the right nostril and blow it out through the mouth. Repeat four to eight times.

▶ The above two exercises are suggested in a laying-down or sitting position, as fresh oxygen can make you light-headed.

▶ Close the mouth. Breathe deep, taking in air through the nostril, blowing air out of the mouth. You can do this while doing strenuous exercise. Otherwise breathe in and out through the nostrils.

▶ The above exercise can be repeated anywhere anytime.

CORRECT THE POSITION OF THE STOMACH

A simple exercise to push the stomach back in place.

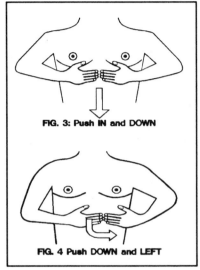

FIG. 3: Push IN and DOWN

FIG. 4 Push DOWN and LEFT

FIGURE 1: Repositioning the Stomach

▶ Place the fingertips of both hands where the ribs come together between the breasts. Pressing fingertips in 1 to 2-1/2 inches, pull or push fingertips all the way down to the belly button. This area may be tender. Repeat 10-12 times.

▶ Next, place fingertips of both hands at the same starting point, between breast where ribs come together, pulling or pushing downward and around the left side, as though you are putting the stomach under the left ribs. Repeat 10-12 times.

▶ This exercise can be done sitting up, lying down, or standing.

ABDOMEN

▶ For *Constipation:* With the tips of all four fingers on both hands, start from the navel (belly button) and rub small circles to the right, progressively increasing the circles diameter to 21 circles.

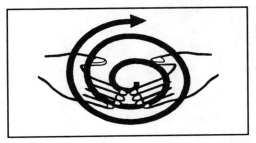

▶ For *Diarrhea:* Repeat the above to the left.

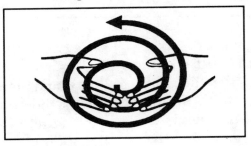

FIGURE 2: The Abdomen

LIFTING THE COLON

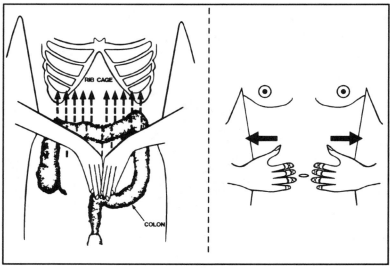

FIGURE 3: Lifting the Colon

► 1. Laying on your back, with the back of your hands together, run fingertips with slight pressure from pelvis to rib cage, beginning in the center of pelvis and making 5 runs upward on each side.

► 2. With all four fingers, start at the belly button and press and pull across the abdomen to each side. Repeat 10 times.

FINGERNAILS

▶ Briskly rub fingernails together. Do this for a few seconds to increase circulation and growth. Repeat the above with thumbnails.

FINGER BRUSHING

▶ Brush the fingertips and fingernails with a nail brush from side to side repeatedly. Can also be done while bathing or washing hands. Very good for removing germs.

FOUR-WAY STRETCH

For a small waist:
▶ Stand upright, arms relaxed at sides. Slowly lean to right until you feel a pull or tightness in waist. Repeat to the left.

▶ Put hands on hips, thumbs forward. Lean upper body back. Return to upright position.

▶ From waist, lean forward, letting relaxed arms dangle. Return to upright position.

▶ Tighten buttocks. For support, stand in open doorway or in hallway – open right hand on the wall, left foot firmly on the floor. Together – swing left stiff arm forward until fingertips point to ceiling and swing right stiff leg back. You will feel a tightness in the buttocks. Do this 8 to 10 times. Repeat using left hand on wall swinging right arm and left leg, 8 to 10 times.

MEN'S CHEST – WOMEN'S BREAST

▶ With right hand, grasp the inside of the left wrist and with left hand, grasp the inside of the right wrist. Lift arms about chin level. Pull clasped wrists toward the chin as though you were trying to make your elbows touch. You will feel the pull in chest muscles.

▶ With the left hand, grasp the inside of the right wrist and with right hand, grasp the inside of the left wrist. Repeat as above.

FACE AND NECK LYMPH

▶ To move lymph, keep shoulders straight and say yes with your head. Move head up and down. Look over right shoulder. Turn head and look over left shoulder. Slowly repeat 10 to 12 times.

▶ Massage when stiff or sore.

~ APPENDIX B ~

SEMINAR NOTES

DIVISION OF THE BODY

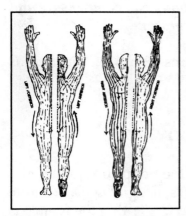

When God saw that Adam had no one or no creation to help him, He put Adam to sleep and out of Adam He created woman. He took a rib, which is half of Adam, and He created woman. And to our knowledge, which hasn't been proven differently to this day, we are divided in half. It's almost as though one side of the body doesn't belong to the other side.

NEUROLOGICAL FUNCTION OF THE BRAIN

Neurologically, we are divided in half. The nerves of the *right* brain works with the *left* side of the body — the nerves of the *left* brain works with the *right* side of the body. It has been proven by medical research that when a stroke occurs, it is as though there is a mark right down the middle of the body. The majority of strokes are caused from a blood flow or nerve default in the brain.

For instance, if *a massive stroke occurs in a particular area* in the left side of the brain *it could* paralyze the right side of the body and one could not talk. The human being talks dominantly from the left side of the brain. If one has a massive stroke in a particular area on the right side of the brain, then *it could* paralyze the left side of the body and one could talk. The body is intelligent. ***The mind and the body can compensate and overrule any diagnostic or symptom.***

Like David said in Psalms 139:14, ..."*the body is fearfully and wonderfully made."*

THE BODY

In discussing the body, the Scripture quotes in 1 Peter 3:7, "*Likewise, ye husbands. . . . giving honour unto the wife, as unto the weaker vessel. . . .*" , that the female is the weaker vessel. The left side of the body is a bit weaker and cooler. Sometimes the nurse taking your blood pressure will take it in one arm and it will register differently when taken in the other. The right side I call the male side of the body. The left side I call the female side. The right side of the body is the positive side, and the left side the negative side — just as you have a positive and a negative current in an electrical wire or a positive and a negative post on a battery. It has been proven that when the electrical forces in our body are balanced, vitality and health are produced.

In the division of the body internally, all organs are much the same in the male and the female. The brain is at the top of the head and the eyes, lungs, heart, stomach, etc., are located in the same place. Internally we are the same with the exception of the reproductive organs. You can take a female heart and transplant it into a male and it will function. The opposite is also true. Blood, if the type is compatible, can also be interchanged.

We are divided in half. We have two brains — the right side and the left side. We have two eyes and two ears. The embryo in the womb before six weeks gestation, has two nostrils on the side of the head. They will eventually come together and make the nose with two nostrils when the baby is maturing in the womb. *Dominantly*, the right nostril oxygenates and nurtures the right side of the brain. The left nostril dominately oxygenates and nurtures the left side of the brain.

When God created Adam, He breathed into the nostrils the breath of life. When we are balanced, we will breath through both sides of the nostrils at the same time. Without that balance the body's intelligence has to compensate. When you breath through the nostrils, you get the oxygen to the brain and it distributes it throughout the body. When you breath through the mouth, it has to get into the lungs, into the bloodstream and then back to the brain. I once was employed in a mental institution. I noticed the majority of retarded people breathed with their mouths open. *Breathe through the nose, you have health and well being. If you breathe through the mouth, you have sickness and disease.* I want to bring to your remembrance that oxygen is our first nutrient. Oxygen has to be in every fiber of the body and its organs.

Continuing through the body, the tongue has different functions, taste, etc. The neck is neutral. Everything that passes from the top of the head to the body, neurologically, will travel through the neck. We have two arms, two rib cages, two lungs, two thymus, two thyroids. We have a thyroid and a parathyroid on each side of the body. We have two chambers in the heart. One side of the heart has a totally different completion than the other side.

Everything that was created on the right side of the body is to remain on the right side of the body. The same on the left side.

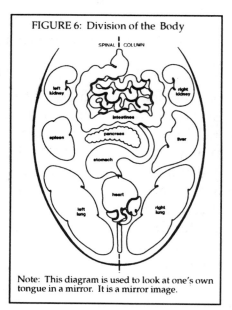

FIGURE 6: Division of the Body

Note: This diagram is used to look at one's own tongue in a mirror. It is a mirror image.

Any time it crosses over that mid-line, physical problems will occur. Where the stomach empties, the first seven to ten inches out of the stomach is on the right side of the body. The stomach is on the left and under the bottom of the left rib. Leaving the stomach, those first seven to ten inches are on the right side. Sometimes those get misplaced from their location. (*Refer to displaced stomach.*) <u>**Every part of the body has an original location**</u> and it must stay in that location if we are going to have good health.

The six feet of the colon that extends from the small intestines to the rectum, has two sides. The right side works differently from the left. When the food enters the right side of the colon (called the ascending colon) just above where the appendix is located through the ileocecal valve, it goes against gravity and travels back up to the rib cage. It does totally different when it gets to the mid-line (the transverse colon) and goes down and out on the left (the descending colon).

We have the liver and the gall bladder on the right side of the body (although part of the liver distinctively extends to the left side). Across the body on the left side, we have a pancreas and the spleen. Going on through the body, you have the two ovaries, the two testicles, two legs, and two feet. When the body has one organ on a particular side, the function of that organ is critical for life — such as the liver on the right side of the body — the pancreas on the left side of the body.

We can live without a gall bladder on the right side of the body or a spleen on the left side. Other organs compensate for the removal of such. We have no substitute for the removal of the liver or pancreas, as opposed to the removal of a kidney or both ovaries.

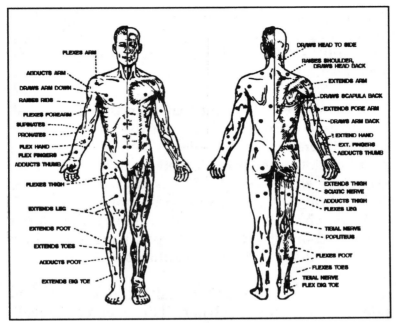

FIGURE 4: Motor Point Chart

The main anatomical parts of the body are:

1. Head
2. Spine
3. Trunk
4. Extremities

The head is subdivided into:

1. Cranium - the top side and back of the skull containing the brain.
2. Face - the front and lower part of the skull including the eyes, nose and mouth.

The spine is a column of bones which supports the head and trunk and protects the spinal cord.

The trunk is subdivided into:

1.   Thorax or Chest - the upper part of the trunk contains the lungs, heart, esophagus or food tube, and part of the trachea or windpipe.

2.   Abdomen - situated below the diaphragm and includes the stomach, intestines, liver and kidneys.

3.   Pelvis - located below the abdomen and contains the rectum, bladder and reproductive organs.

The extremities include:

1.   Upper limbs - shoulder, arm, forearm and hand.

2.   Lower limbs - thigh, leg and foot.

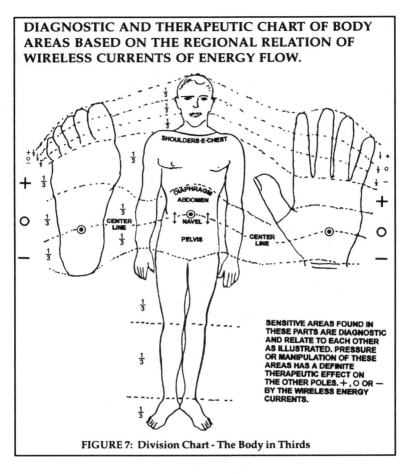

**DIAGNOSTIC AND THERAPEUTIC CHART OF BODY
AREAS BASED ON THE REGIONAL RELATION OF
WIRELESS CURRENTS OF ENERGY FLOW.**

SENSITIVE AREAS FOUND IN THESE PARTS ARE DIAGNOSTIC AND RELATE TO EACH OTHER AS ILLUSTRATED. PRESSURE OR MANIPULATION OF THESE AREAS HAS A DEFINITE THERAPEUTIC EFFECT ON THE OTHER POLES. +, O OR − BY THE WIRELESS ENERGY CURRENTS.

FIGURE 7: Division Chart - The Body in Thirds

The body is also divided into thirds *horizontally.*
We've pretty well covered what consists of the body
dividing in half. If you can visualize the body divided
into thirds, these divisions are distinctively marked in
the body. They are not thirds as equals, but thirds as in
quotations. From the top of the head to the eye is a
third. From the eye to the mouth is a third. The chin is
a third. The neck is neutral.

Head:
> Top of the head to the eyes is a third.
> Eyes to the mouth is a third.
> Chin is a third.

Torso:
> Shoulder to the rib cage is a third.
> Rib cage to the hip is a third
> And the pelvis is a third.

Arms:
> Shoulder to the elbow is a third.
> Elbow to the wrist is a third.
> The hand is a third.

Legs:
> Hip to the knee is a third.
> Knee to the ankle is a third.
> Foot is a third.

Diagnostic. If you hurt — what side is hurting? Is it hurting on the right side? Is it hurting in the middle? Is it hurting on the left? Try to narrow it to what side of the body, what third of the body. And just visualize what organ or body function is located in that area. This will give you a general idea. If the symptom persists, see your doctor.

One of my own diagnoses is when I awake in the morning, I bend my fingers. I take note which hand, which finger is stiff. When stiff, I know that the day before I have taken in foods that consist of too much acid or I've been under extreme stress which produces acid.

DIAGNOSIS —— MEDICAL, PHYSICAL AND SPIRITUAL

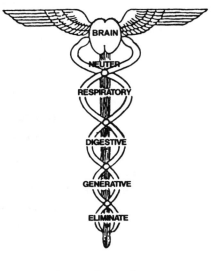

The doctor's emblem, the medical emblem which is called the caduceus, consists of the two wings, the rod and the serpents winding up the rod. When you see this emblem, you know there is medical involved. You see this emblem on all prescriptions, hospitals, etc. The emblem with just one serpent on it, such as the one you see associated with a chiropractor or on an ambulance, indicates that they are assisting the body, but not prescribing for it. The origination of the right and left wing represents the right and left hemisphere of the brain. And the staff represents the backbone of the body. And the serpents, (which have nothing to do with snakes) represent wireless electric currents that are the life force that weaves in and out of the body.

▶ *Medical doctors* have different ways of analyzing what is going on within the body. For instance, the hair tells what is going on in the body. Taking samples of the blood, urine, feces (which is the bowel), and spit (the saliva in the mouth), can provide invaluable information. In so doing they can determine what is going on within the body. Also the use of electrical equipment such as EKG, MRI, EEG, sonogram, etc., can determine the condition of the physical body.

▶ *Chiropractors* analyze the vertebrae of the backbone, from the base of the skull to the tip of your tailbone. They will correlate the nerves that go to a particular organ or function of the body. By analyzing the spine they can diagnose what is going on in the body using these points.

▶ *Reflexologists* can determine in the feet all points that reflect the body. All diagnostic points in the body can be detected in the hands, fingers, tongue, ears and face.

▶ *Iridologists* will analyze the eyes to see what's going on in the body.

▶ *Acupuncturists* will go by the points in the ears and entire body.

Another way of analyzing the body is the *colon*. A narrow or balloon point in the colon can point to dysfunction in the body.

There are two kinds of drugs — those that sedate and those that stimulate. ***Balance is the key***. When the body is overactive, you want to slow that down, sedate it. When it's underactive you want to stimulate it to its original balance. Sometimes a doctor will prescribe a drug. Sometimes a food supplement is given. A supplement is something that supplies what that particular part of the body is not supplying on its own. That's why vitamins, if they are derived from food or natural source are called supplements. Foods do the same thing. Foods can either sedate or stimulate. Live foods stimulate and sedate plus feed the body. Some drugs will just stimulate an organ to get that organ to work on its own.

PHYSICAL

We have physical symptoms that will let us know the cause. We have a tendency to sedate the symptom instead of eliminating the cause.

The Body Talks – What is it Saying?

▶ Hair

If the hair is unhealthy, so is the body. Is the hair brittle? Dry? Breaks easily? Is hair oily? Thick or Thin?

Matthew 10:30 — *"But the very hairs of your head are all numbered."*

▶ Ears

Are the ear lobes equal in color? Are they extra white or extra red? Stand out at top or bottom?

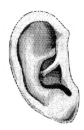

Proverbs 15:31,32 — *"The ear that heareth the reproof of life abideth among the wise. He that refuseth instruction despiseth his own soul; but he that heareth reproof getteth understanding."*

▶ Eyes

Is shape the same or is one large, one small? Is one higher than the other? Is one pupil or iris larger than the other? Which one?

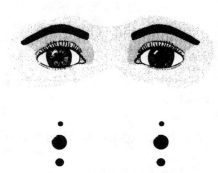

▶ Mouth

Are lips narrow or thick? Top lip larger? Top lip smaller? Corners turned up or down? One side of top or bottom lip smaller? One side only droops? Swollen – does it swell & where is the swelling? Is it just at times? Cracked or bleeding? Creases at top or bottom?

▶ These are symptoms - where is the cause?

▶ Tongue

Coated? Where? What color?

Cracked? Where and what directions or pattern does crack follow?

Creased? Straight? Down Center? Does it go all the way? Crooked crease? Like a River?

Full? Does it fill the mouth? Too full?

Flexible? Long? Easy to stick tongue out?

Short? Easy to retract?

Teeth prints on tongue? Where? On side? Front?

Roll? Can you curve each side of tongue up (roll tongue)?

Stick to the roof of mouth?

Is the color even? Purplish red or shining? Blotched: under tongue, purple, blue red? NOT TO WORRY.

Proverbs 18:21 — *"Death and life are in the power of the tongue; and they that love it shall eat the fruit thereof."*

SPIRITUAL

We have a physical body and a spiritual body. What we put in the physical body is what we become physically. What we put into the spiritual body is what we become spiritually. Proverbs 23:7 says, *"For as he thinketh in his heart, so is he..."* This is speaking to the spiritual heart, not the one physical that's divided in half. *"From the abundance of the heart, the mouth speaketh"* (Matthew 12:34) ... this is the spiritual body.

Without the physical heart, the body could not exist. In the womb we become a physical and a spiritual body. At birth when we take in that *breath of life* which God breathed into Adam, we become a living soul, a living heart. We breathe and continue to hear, see, touch, smell, feel, taste and breathe. Whatever situation we are put in, or we put ourselves in, determines our physical as well as our spiritually. ***It's not what comes our way, but how we handle it***. This is the motto that I survive by. "It's not what comes my way, but how I handle it."

JEANNIE CALLIS, a Mentor of Health,
teaches groups, organizations, churches, families, and anyone interested in improving their health.

THIS INFORMATION COULD CHANGE YOUR LIFE.

To set up or attend a class
WRITE:

JEANNIE CALLIS
P. O. BOX 152
ARGYLE, TEXAS 76226
1-800-752-5313

~ APPENDIX C ~

NOTES

▶ I am repeatedly asked about my age and high energy level. My reply is: age 65. Energy: I watch my stress level and my acid food intake.

▶ The personal vitamin that I take is Vitacel 7. The cost is at this time is $16 for a bottle of 60 tablets. I have found that I have more energy, enhanced eyesight, improved sleep patterns, a sense of well-being. I have also noticed the symptoms of depression are eliminated. I have also had a restoration of my thinning hair. I have watched my hair color restored. For information about this product call Nutritional Engineering, Ltd. 1-800-225-6799, using code # 5020.

▶ *Here's a special message to you - - - - -*

Hugs

It's wondrous what a hug can do,
A hug can cheer you when you're blue.
A hug can say, "I love you so,"
or, "Gee! I hate to see you go."
A hug is, "Welcome back again!"
and, "Great to see you!" or
"Where've you been?"

A hug can soothe a small child's pain
and bring a rainbow after rain.

The hug! There's just no doubt about it,
We scarcely could survive without it.
A hug delights and warms and charms,
It must be why God gave us arms.

Hugs are great for fathers and mothers,
sweet for sisters, swell for brothers,
and chances are some favorite aunts
love them more than potted plants.

Kittens crave them. Puppies love them.
Heads of state are not above them.
A hug can break the language barrier,
and make the dullest day seem merrier.

No need to fret about the store of 'em.
The more you give, the more there are of 'em.
So stretch those arms without delay
and give someone a hug today.

Author Unknown

~ APPENDIX D ~

ORDER FORMS

COLEMA™ BOARD - $165.00
(includes shipping and handling)

Number of Boards: _____ x $165 = $_____
Extra Tips ($3.00 Each) _____ x $ 3 = $_____

Total Amount Enclosed $_____

Name: _____
Address: _____
_____
City: _____
State: _____ Zip:_____
Phone: (_____)_____

Please send check or money order to:

Jeannie Callis
P. O. Box 152
Argyle, Texas 76226
1-800-752-5313

JEANNIE CALLIS
P. O. BOX 152 • ARGYLE, TEXAS 76226
1-800-752-5313

DATE:_____

ORDER FORM

CUSTOMER INFORMATION:
Name: _____
Address: _____
_____ZIP_____
Phone: _____

SHIP TO:
Name: _____
Address: _____
_____ZIP_____
Phone: _____

No. of Units	Item	Units per Case	Unit Price	Total Amount
	"16" Detoxificant, 1 qt.	12	9.50	
	"19" Intestinal Cleanser, 10 oz.	6	13.00	
	"19A" Herb Tablet, 100 tabs.	12	12.00	
	"22S" GREENLIFE , 360 tabs.	12	25.50	
	"48" Beet Juice, 150 tabs.	12	15.50	
	"53S" Wheat Germ Oil, 120 caps.	12	10.00	
	"54S" Enzymatic Supplement, 100 tabs.	12	11.00	
			Sub-Total	
	*Shipping Charges (Add 10% of the Sub-Total/ Not less than $5.00)			
	TOTAL – CHECK OR MONEY ORDER ONLY			

To contact the author, write:
Jeannie Callis
P. O. Box 152
Argyle, Texas 76226
1-800-752-5313

Additional copies of this book, *Temple Talk Volume #1*,
are available for $10.00 (plus $2.50 shipping and
handling) by completing the following form and
mailing along with a check or money order to:

Jeannie Callis
P. O. Box 152
Argyle, Texas 76226

Name: _____
Address:_____
_____
City: _____
State: _____ Zip:_____
Phone: (_____)_____